The Menopause and Hormone Replacement Therapy
Second Edition

D1643374

The Menopause and Hormone Replacement Therapy
Second Edition

Roger N J Smith, MRCP MRCOG
Consultant Obstetrician and Gynaecologist
Queen Mary's Hospital
Sidcup
Kent, UK

John W W Studd, DSc MD FRCOG
Consultant Gynaecologist
The Chelsea and Westminster Hospital
Fulham Road
London, UK

Supported by an educational grant from
Janssen-Cilag Ltd

MARTIN DUNITZ

Although every effort has been made to ensure that the drug doses and other information are presented accurately in this publication, the ultimate responsibility rests with the prescribing physician. Neither the publishers nor the authors nor Janssen-Cilag can be held responsible for errors or for any other consequences arising from the use of information contained herein.

The opinions expressed in this book are those of the authors and do not necessarily reflect those of Janssen-Cilag.

© Martin Dunitz Ltd 1993, 1998

First published in the United Kingdom
in 1993 by
Martin Dunitz Ltd
7–9 Pratt Street
London NW1 0AE

Reprinted 1994
Second edition 1998

ISBN 1-85317-620-6

Printed and bound in Spain by Cayfosa

Contents

Introduction 1

Climacteric and
menopausal symptoms 3

The long-term health implications
of the menopause and HRT 10

Complications of HRT 32

Routes of administration of HRT 42

Practical notes on prescribing HRT 48

References 58

Index 62

John Studd is Consultant Gynaecologist at the Chelsea and Westminster Hospital, London. He started the first menopause clinic in the UK in Birmingham, and his team were the first to quantify the protective effect of progestogens on the endometrium and show the beneficial effects of oestrogens on pre-menstrual depression and post-natal depression. He was Consultant Gynaecologist at King's College Hospital, London for 20 years, and is director of the Fertility and Endocrinology Centre at the Lister Hospital, London. He has published over 400 original papers on reproductive medicine and is the author or editor of 24 books on post-graduate obstetrics and gynaecology. At the Chelsea and Westminster Hospital, he runs the Menopause Clinic, Premenstrual Syndrome Clinic and a Psycho-endocrine Clinic: this last clinic is a new concept and will investigate many of the emotional and endocrine problems of women.

Roger Smith is Consultant Obstetrician and Gynaecologist at Queen Mary's Hospital, Sidcup, Kent. He qualified in Manchester undertaking general professional training in both General Medicine and Obstetrics and Gynaecology. After registrar training at Queen Charlotte's & Chelsea Hospital, he joined Mr Studd as clinical research fellow from 1991 to 1994, working with him at both King's College Hospital and the Chelsea and Westminster Hospital, persuing research interests in menopause and premenstrual syndrome. He then joined the King's College Hospital Senior Registrar rotation working principally for Professor Linda Cardozo, prior to taking up his Consultant appointment in June 1997. His current interests are: menopause, urogynaecology and high risk obstetrics.

Introduction

The term menopause refers specifically to the cessation of menstruation, which occurs at an average age of 51 years in developed countries. It is the most obvious manifestation of a gradual decline in ovarian function which commences about 5 years before a woman's last period. The ovaries fail because they run out of primordial follicles. Initially, this results in increasingly frequent failure of ovulation, together with a compensatory increase in gonadotrophin secretion in an effort to maintain hormone levels. Despite this, hormone production declines progressively. In the short term, these falling oestrogen levels commonly result in a spectrum of unpleasant symptoms such as flushes, sweats, vaginal dryness and depression.

The term climacteric refers to this whole involutional era which commonly spans 5 years each side of the menopause. In the long term, absolute oestrogen deficiency leads to a generalized atrophy of the skin, an accelerated rate of bone loss from the skeleton producing osteoporosis, and a rapid increase in the incidence of coronary heart disease. All of these adverse sequelae may potentially be reversed by hormone replacement therapy (HRT).

In developed countries, the average woman lives one-third or more of her life after the menopause, and climacteric and post-menopausal woman constitute 20% of the entire population (Figure 1). It is difficult to know how many climacteric women do receive HRT, but the numbers appear to be increasing. A recent population-based survey in Scotland found that 19% of women aged 45–54 were current users of HRT (Porter *et al.*, 1996). It is likely that this figure declines rapidly with advancing age.

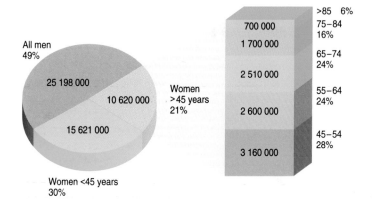

Figure 1
Number of climacteric and post-menopausal women in England and Wales. (From Office of Population Censuses and Statistics Cause 1993, series DH2, No. 20. London HMSO, 1994.)

Classic menopause symptoms

Hot flushes, night sweats, sleep disturbance and vaginal dryness are the 'classic' menopause symptoms. Few would dispute that they peak in incidence during the climacteric years and that they are caused by the hormonal changes of declining ovarian function. Cross-sectional population-based data indicate that they are common in that 84% of women experience at least one classic menopause symptom (Porter *et al.*, 1996). Although many women are not particularly distressed by such symptoms, 45% describe them as problematic. When hot flushes are experienced, they occur daily or more frequently in 70% of women, lead to embarrassment in 70%, cause acute physical distress in 50%, and persist for more than 5 years in 25% (McKinley and Jefferys, 1974). Although such classic menopause symptoms occur most frequently in the year immediately following the last period, it is important to remember that they are still common in premenopausal climacteric women in whom periods may still be regular although the gonadotrophin levels are not usually elevated.

3

Classic menopause symptoms	

Symptoms:	Occurrence:
• Hot flushes	• Affect 80% of women
• Sweats	• Problematic in 45% of women
• Sleep disturbances	
• Vaginal dryness	• Last more than 5 years in 25%

 # *Vasomotor symptoms*

Flushes and sweats result from vasomotor instability and are associated with increased skin temperature, decreased skin conductivity, sweating and feelings of faintness. They disturb sleep and may also cause giddiness. The latter may be responsible for the increased incidence of falls in women in their 60s compared with men. Headache, another common symptom of the menopause, is also thought to be of vasomotor origin. The precise cause of this central and peripheral vasomotor instability is unknown. Declining oestrogen levels are important but elevated gonadotrophin levels are not.

The dosage levels employed in commonly used HRT preparations were determined on the basis of relief of vasomotor symptoms. Thus, low-to-moderate dose HRT is highly effective in the abolition of sweats and flushes. Clonidine may partially relieve vasomotor symptoms but is very inferior to oestrogen. In the rare cases in which oestrogen is contraindicated, high dose progestogen may also provide some relief from hot flushes and sweats.

Genital atrophy and urinary symptoms

Vaginal dryness results from lack of normal secretions consequent on atrophy of the vaginal skin, and is associated with an increased incidence of infections such as candidiasis. This is atrophic vaginitis. The resultant dyspareunia will frequently lead to a secondary loss of libido. Similar atrophy of the oestrogen-sensitive mucosa of the urethra and trigone may contribute to the high incidence of urinary symptoms, such as incontinence, frequency, urgency and dysuria, seen in climacteric and post-menopausal women. Low-to-moderate dose HRT will reverse genital atrophy and relieve vaginal dryness, dyspareunia and secondary loss of libido. Effects upon urinary function are less certain. Clinical experience indicates that HRT reduces the incidence of urinary sensory dysfunction such as recurrent cystitis, urgency and frequency, and may also reduce the frequency of urinary tract infections, but there is not a clear improvement in urinary stress incontinence (Cardozo and Kelleher, 1997).

Symptoms of urogenital atrophy

• Vaginal dryness	• Urinary urgency
• Dyspareunia	• Urinary frequency
• Atrophic vaginitis	• Vaginal discharge
• 'Cystitis'	• Vaginal bleeding

Psychological symptoms

More controversial is the contention that declining ovarian function gives rise to a spectrum of psychological symptoms. Certainly depression, irritability, loss of confidence, poor memory, poor concentration and primary loss of libido are common complaints of women attending menopause clinics and may be severe. It seems intuitively reasonable to assume that the end result of repeated sleep disturbance by nocturnal flushes and sweats is likely to be precisely these psychological symptoms. Some studies have found such symptoms to peak in incidence in women aged 45–55 years, although other workers have found no such relationship to the menopause (Bungay *et al.*, 1980).

The debate as to whether the hormonal changes of the menopause are directly responsible for psychological symptoms is perhaps academic. Undoubtedly, psychological symptoms are common in women in the climacteric decade. A population-based survey found that 51% of women in this age group reported depression in the preceding 6 months and 22% described the depression as a significant problem, whilst a standard self-reporting measure of depression (Centre for Epidemiological Studies Depression Scale) rated 30% of this population as depressed (Porter *et al.*, 1996). Therefore, whatever the underlying cause, depression is clearly a significant health issue in climacteric women. It is likely that the other psychological symptoms reported are at least exacerbated by depressed mood.

An aetiological role for the sex steroids in climacteric depression is supported by the occurrence of similar symptoms at other times of hormonal flux, such as post-natal depression and pre-menstrual syndrome, and by the excellent response of such symptoms to hormone replacement observed in many women (Smith *et al.*, 1995; Gregoire *et al.*, 1996). This has led to the concept of a triad of oestrogen-responsive mood disorders which are often inter-related as a continuum in the same patient: (i) post-natal depression; (ii) pre-menstrual depression; and (iii) climacteric depression (Studd and Smith, 1994).

Psychological symptoms

- Depression
- Irritability
- Poor memory
- Difficulty concentrating
- Loss of confidence
- Loss of energy
- Panic attacks
- Loss of libido

It is relevant to differentiate between depressed mood and a clinical depressive illness. There are considerable data from randomized trials to indicate that oestrogen can elevate mood (Smith and Studd, 1994). Ditkoff *et al.* (1991) found that standard doses of oral oestrogen elevated mood scores in women who were not clinically depressed. In another trial, moderately high doses of oestrogen, achieved with 50 mg subcutaneous implants of oestradiol, resulted in significant reductions in depression scores compared with placebo; the improvement compared with baseline still being evident after nearly 2 years (Montgomery *et al.*, 1987). This effect was, however, confined to premenopausal climacteric women. This suggests that perhaps there is a distinct climacteric depression which is confined to women undergoing the most marked hormonal changes.

In a remarkable study by Klaiber *et al.* (1979), much higher supraphysiological doses of oestrogen have been found to have significant antidepressant effects in women with severe depressive illness unresponsive to conventional therapy. Given our current understanding of the interaction between oestrogens and central neurotransmitter mechanisms, these mood regulating and antidepressant effects of oestrogen should come as no surprise. Oestrogen administration increases activity in a number of central nervous system neurotransmitter systems, but particularly in the serotoninergic system. (Perhaps we should come to regard oestrogen as a naturally occurring antidepressant)

Once women have traversed the turmoil of the climacteric years and reached the hormonal steady-state of the post-menopause there is almost certainly no increase in the incidence of depression. In fact, many women experience considerable improvement in general well-being after their periods stop, because of loss of cyclical headaches, PMS, dysmenorrhoea and bleeding.

There is a high incidence of psychiatric illness amongst women attending a menopause clinic, but a menopause clinic is a biased population as many women with climacteric or endogenous depression will attend hoping that oestrogens are effective. These women need skilled counselling and treatment.

Libido

(Primary loss of libido occurring during the climacteric can be attributed to androgen deficiency) Data indicate that testosterone is involved in the modulation of sexual drive in premenopausal women, and androgen levels decline by half as a consequence of loss of ovarian production after the menopause. The administration of subcutaneous implants of 100 mg testosterone will restore libido in 80% of climacteric women. A 100 mg testosterone implant releases between 0.35 and 1 mg of testosterone per day during its 6 month life-span. This dosage elevates testosterone back to the upper end of the normal premenopausal range and, when given in combination with oestradiol implants, has little impact on lipids (Studd and Smith, 1993). Unfortunately, the new transdermal testosterone delivery system, the Andropatch (SmithKline Beecham), delivers too high a dose of testosterone (2.5 mg per day) to be recommended for use in women. Oral androgen preparations containing methyltestosterone cannot be recommended because of adverse hepatic effects.

Generalized atrophy and aches and pains

During and after the menopause there is a generalized loss of collagen from skin, muscle and bone. This results in thin skin and the generalized musculoskeletal aches and pains so frequently experienced by climacteric women. Such symptoms respond well to HRT. Furthermore, oestrogen also increases both skin collagen content, skin thickness (Brincat *et al.*, 1985) and collagen in the bone matrix.

Generalized atrophy of connective tissues

- Skin thinning
- Osteoporosis
- Generalized aches and pains
- Loss of hair
- Brittle nails
- Bone pain

Osteoporosis

Osteoporosis is defined as a state in which bone is normally mineralized but reduced in quantity, resulting in bones which are weaker and thus more prone to fracture. Bone density in both sexes peaks in the third decade, then gradually declines, but in women the rate of bone loss accelerates substantially with the menopause such that bone density decreases by 2% per annum in the spine and 1% in the hip. By the age of 60, 25% of Caucasian women have radiological evidence of vertebral crush fractures (Stevenson and Whitehead, 1982). Women lose 50% of their total skeleton by the age of 70, whereas men lose only 25% by the age of 90.

While such spinal osteoporosis results in loss of height, pain, deformity and the typical 'dowagers hump', it is fracture of the femoral neck which puts the greatest strain on health care resources. The annual incidence of hip fracture rises from 0.07 per 1000 women aged 35–40 years to 29.1 per 1000 in those aged 85 or over. In the United States, this translates into 300 000 femoral neck fractures per year, increasing at a rate of 10 000–20 000 annually as the population ages, whilst in the UK there are currently 60 000 femoral neck fractures annually. Worryingly, there is some evidence that the age-adjusted incidence of hip fracture is increasing, meaning that this escalating prevalence is not only due to demographic changes, but may also reflect a deteriorating quality of bone in today's elderly women (Kannus *et al.*, 1995). <u>Once a hip fracture has occurred it results in death within 12 months in 20%</u> and <u>permanent loss of social independence in 50%</u>. The financial costs are enormous and increase every year; currently they amount to £942 million per year in the UK.

There is a clear causal relationship between oestrogen deficiency, as seen following menopause, and a change in bone metabolism, resulting in a progressive decline in bone density and an increasing incidence of clinically relevant osteoporosis. This not only pertains to the post-menopausal years but to any situation in which prolonged oestrogen deficiency occurs. This applies to premature menopause and also to oligo- or amenorrhoea of any cause, with polycystic ovary syndrome being the one most commonly encountered in clinical practice.

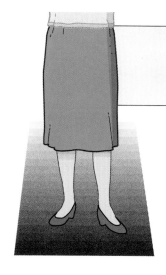

HRT given for 5 years halves the lifetime risk of hip fracture

Hormonal treatment

Oestrogen replacement must be regarded as the benchmark against which all treatments aimed at reducing the burden of osteoporosis must be judged. It has been clearly shown that oestrogen replacement, even in low doses, prevents further loss of bone from the skeleton and thus arrests the osteoporotic process, resulting in a reduced risk of fracture (Keil *et al.*, 1987). Indeed, most of the oestrogen preparations used currently actually cause a modest increase in bone density, at least in the first few years of therapy. The magnitude of this effect is dose dependent. Oral therapy, the least potent form,

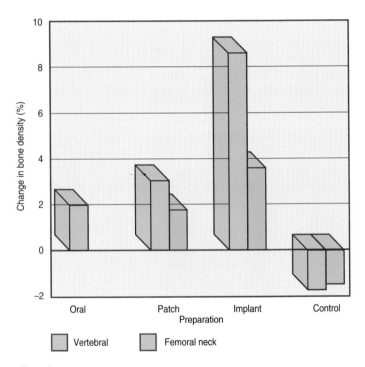

Figure 2
Annual increment in bone density with different routes of oestrogen administration. Doses: implant, 75 mg; patch, 50 µg; oral, 2 mg.

increases bone density by ~2% per annum in the lumbar spine, a 50 μg percutaneous patch achieves a 3.5% increment, but the greatest effect is seen with oestradiol implants, the most potent form of oestrogen administration, which bring about an 8.4% increase in vertebral bone density per year (Figure 2) (Lindsay *et al.*, 1976; Christiansen and Christiansen, 1981; Stevenson *et al.*, 1990; Studd *et al.*, 1990). The data demonstrate a significant positive correlation between blood oestradiol levels and the incremental increase in both vertebral and femoral neck bone density. Reduction in fracture risk is also dependent upon duration of therapy. Five years of low dose oral therapy reduces the lifetime incidence of femoral neck fracture by 50%.

Ideally, all post-menopausal women should be screened for osteoporosis risk by means of a bone density scan. The knowledge that she has a low bone density may persuade a woman to use HRT and also helps the physician assess the dose and route of administration necessary.

Non-hormonal treatment
Much effort has been expended in the search for non-hormonal methods of preventing osteoporosis. While exercise certainly has an impact upon peak adult bone mass it does not prevent osteoporosis. Similarly, while a diet deficient in calcium may predispose to low bone density, dietary calcium supplements in those with a normal dietary intake are probably of no clinical value. Calcitonin reduces the rate of bone loss but so far has not been demonstrated to reduce fracture risk. The injectable form is expensive and unpopular with patients while the intranasal preparation is even more expensive.

The importance of demonstrating a clinical reduction in fracture rates is well illustrated by fluoride. While increasing spinal bone density, it has actually been found to increase the risk of non-vertebral fractures, highlighting the fact that quality of bone is as important as density.

Bisphosphonates

The most promising non-hormonal group of compounds for the treatment of osteoporosis are the bisphosphonates. Etidronate was the first commercially available. Studies confirmed its ability to increase bone density (by 2% per annum in the lumbar spine) and there are also data showing that it can reduce the incidence of radiologically detected vertebral fractures. Alendronate is a newer compound which has the advantage of a simplified schedule of administration. The optimal dose of alendronate is 10 mg daily, which has been shown to increase bone mineral density by an average of 3.2% annually over a 3-year period at the lumbar spine, with corresponding increases of 1.6% at the femoral neck and 2.5% at the trochanter. A recently published meta-analysis of five studies provides evidence that not only does alendronate increase bone density, but that it also has a clinically important effect in reducing fracture rates over a 2-year period, with a relative risk of non-vertebral fractures of 0.71 (95% confidence interval, 0.5–0.99) compared with placebo (Karpf *et al.*, 1997). In general, alendronate is well tolerated, but it will cause abdominal pain in some women, although this usually settles with continued use.

These early data with etidronate and alendronate are encouraging, but there is a need for long-term data on fracture rates. At present, oestrogen replacement must be considered to be the first-line therapy for prevention and remedial treatment of established osteopaenia. In the rare circumstances where there exists a real contraindication to treatment with oestrogen or where the individual has an aversion to oestrogen, alendronate should currently be considered as second-line therapy of choice.

Ischaemic heart disease

At the age of 45, men are 5- to 6-times as likely as women to die from ischaemic heart disease (IHD). After the menopause, however, women rapidly catch up so that, by the age of 60, death rates are equal with IHD thereafter remaining the leading cause of death in both sexes, and increasing exponentially with age (Figure 3). The most likely explanation for this is that oestrogens protect women from IHD prior to menopause.

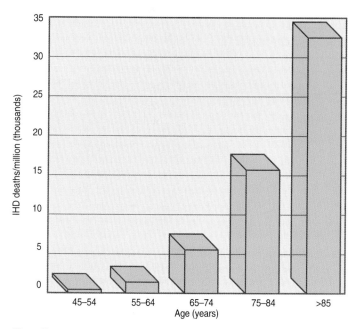

Figure 3
UK annual mortality from ischaemic heart disease (per million). (From Office of Population Censuses and Statistics Cause 1993, series DH2, No. 20. London HMSO, 1994.)

There is now a wealth of convincing data concerning the impact of hormone replacement therapy on IHD. It is one of these rare instances where the data are in agreement. Out of 31 published studies over the past 20 years, only two have failed to find any change in incidence of IHD with HRT, four have found an increased incidence although the differences were not statistically significant, whereas 25 have observed a reduced risk, 12 of which reached statistical significance. Pooling results from all these studies yields a relative risk of IHD of only 0.56 (95% confidence interval, 0.5–0.61) in oestrogen users. Restricting analysis to only those studies with a prospective cohort design with internal controls gives a relative risk of IHD of 0.58 (95% confidence interval, 0.48–0.69) amongst oestrogen users (Stampfer and Colditz, 1991) (Figure 4).

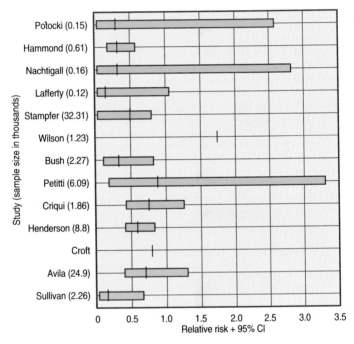

Figure 4
Oestrogen and risk of IHD. CI, confidence interval. [Adapted from Stampfer and Colditz (1991) with permission.]

There are also data from a smaller number of studies to indicate that oestrogen replacement reduces the risk of stroke by ~20% (Paganini-Hill *et al.*, 1988).

These data can be criticized because the studies were not randomized, and it may be that, over the last 20 years, low-risk women have been preferentially given oestrogen. Thus, these optimistic results may be biased. This seems unlikely, however, because the impact of oestrogen is as great if not greater in high-risk women, such as those with hyperlipidaemia, hypertension or previous heart attacks (Bush *et al.*, 1987). It is likely, therefore, that these data do indicate a real reduction in incidence of IHD with HRT. Ideally, a randomized controlled trial of a huge cohort is required but for ethical and practical reasons this is unlikely to happen.

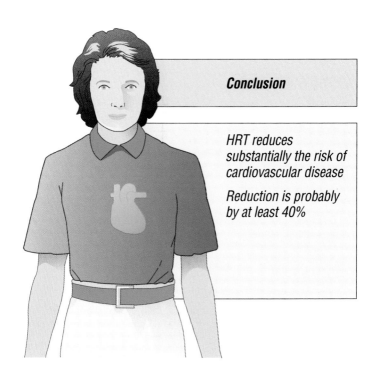

Conclusion

HRT reduces substantially the risk of cardiovascular disease

Reduction is probably by at least 40%

Mechanism of action of oestrogen in IHD

What is the mechanism of action of oestrogen on IHD? In untreated women, after the menopause, LDL cholesterol increases and HDL declines. This is consistent with the general understanding of lipids as risk factors for IHD. Oestrogen replacement partially reverses these unfavourable lipid changes. There is increasing evidence, however, that its actions are more complex than lipid effects alone. Using Doppler colour flow imaging techniques it has been found that blood flow at several sites, including the uterine and carotid arteries, decreases with the menopause, but is restored by oestrogen replacement. Animal studies have shown that oestrogen has a direct effect on the arterial wall by inhibiting the accumulation of cholesterol, the major precursor of atherosclerotic plaques. In addition, oestrogen may act through effects on glucose and fat metabolism. These are both linked to IHD risk and are both modulated by oestrogen. Thus, the clinical experience of oestrogen use and IHD is validated by an increasing body of basic scientific data.

Progestogen in IHD

The bulk of the data on IHD and HRT comes from studies employing oral oestrogen, most often conjugated equine oestrogens, given alone unopposed by progestogen. Current practice dictates that cyclical progestogen should always be prescribed with oestrogen if the woman has a uterus. By them-selves, all progestogens have a tendency to reduce HDL and elevate LDL cholesterol. This has led to the concern that the widespread incorporation of progestogens in HRT might reduce the beneficial cardiovascular effects. The net effect of any combination upon lipids will depend upon the balance between oestrogen and progestogen. Low doses of progesto-gen combined sequentially with oestrogen do have a marginal impact upon lipids, but this is too small to be of clinical signifi-cance. For example, a study in which 43% of oestrogen use was opposed by sequential progestogen still found over a 50% reduction in risk of IHD (Hunt et al., 1990). This is consistent with the realization that, while lipid changes are relevant, they are only part of the story with increased blood flow being of greater importance.

Continuous combined HRT

No studies are as yet available to assess the cardiovascular disease risk associated with 'continuous combined' HRT regimens, but they appear to produce similar lipid changes to sequential HRT. One very recently published study compared the impact of continuous combined HRT with the lipid-lowering drug simvastatin on lipids, in a group of post-menopausal women with hypercholesterolaemia (Darling et al., 1997). The combination of 1.25 mg of conjugated equine oestrogens and 5 mg of medroxyprogesterone acetate daily produced a similar rise in HDL and a similar fall in LDL to simvastatin. Interestingly, the HRT resulted in a 27% fall in Lp(a) lipoprotein levels not seen with simvastatin, and which may be of significance as Lp(a) appears to be an independent risk factor for cardiovascular disease in women. It seems likely therefore that continuous combined HRT regimens will also result in a substantial decrease in IHD.

Summary

It is evident that the data sheets which list IHD, and risk factors for IHD, as contraindications to HRT, are both wrong and dangerously misleading. This misinformation has arisen because of the inaccurate extrapolation of data about synthetic oestrogens in the contraceptive pill. The natural oestrogens employed in HRT are pharmacologically very different from the synthetic oestrogens in the pill.

The data indicate that HRT reduces the risk of IHD even in women at high risk. Therefore, the presence of angina, a previous myocardial infarction, hypertension, hyperlipidaemia, a family history of premature IHD, or indeed any other risk factor for IHD, should be regarded as positive indications for HRT.

Alzheimer's disease

One of the most exciting recent developments is the early data indicating that oestrogen may have beneficial effects in both preventing and ameliorating Alzheimer's disease. On a basic science level there are several possible mechanisms of action:

- Oestrogen is an important co-factor for nerve growth factors
- Oestrogen increases cerebral blood flow
- Oestrogen increases activity in several neurotransmitter systems (with a particularly marked effect on the cholinergic system which is specifically deficient in Alzheimer's disease)
- Oestrogen is able to prevent neuronal atrophy in certain brain areas involved primarily in the pathology of Alzheimer's

On a clinical level, there is evidence that oestrogen improves memory, that women with Alzheimer's are less likely to have taken HRT previously and that administration of a standard dose oral HRT improves mental test scores in women with established Alzheimer's.

The most impressive data, however, come from Tang *et al.* (1996) who, in a large prospective study of 1124 elderly women in New York, found that women who gave a history of past oestrogen use had a significantly reduced risk of developing Alzheimer's disease. The risk of a diagnosis of Alzheimer's being made during the study period in women who had never used oestrogen was 16.3% compared with only 5.8% in never-users of oestrogen and only 1.7% (relative risk, 0.13; 95% confidence interval, 0.02–0.92) in women who had used oestrogen for more than 1 year (average duration of use 13.6 years).

The Tang study is of good quality but its findings need to be confirmed by others. The possibility that the risk of developing Alzheimer's disease can be reduced dramatically by using HRT has far reaching consequences both for the individual in terms of years of good quality life, and also for society in terms of healthcare expenditure on institutional care for the demented elderly.

Oestrogen use and Alzheimer's disease

- Oestrogen may reduce risk of developing Alzheimer's in current HRT users
- Oestrogen may improve cognitive performance in women with established Alzheimer's disease

---

Endometrial hyperplasia and carcinoma

Oestrogen replacement alone, unopposed by progestogen therapy, causes hyperstimulation of the endometrium with an increased risk of both hyperplasia and carcinoma. The risk of carcinoma is related to both the dosage and duration of oestrogen use. Use of unopposed oestrogen for up to 3 years increases risk of endometrial carcinoma by a factor of 9, and 15 or more years use by a factor of 34 to give an annual incidence of 11.8 per 1000 women. Furthermore, the risk only declines slowly and may still be increased 10 years after use of unopposed oestrogen is discontinued. However, oestrogen-induced tumours are usually well differentiated with a high cure rate. The result is that, despite the widespread use of unopposed oestrogen, up until the mid-1970s there was no associated increase in mortality from the disorder.

Hyperplasia is found on biopsy in up to 56% of women receiving long-term unopposed oestrogen. As carcinoma is a progression from atypical hyperplasia, the carcinogenic process can be prevented simply by the administration of progestogen cyclically each month. The degree of protection offered is related directly to the number of days per month for which the progestogen is taken. Ten to thirteen days appears to offer complete protection; thus, most combinations of oestrogen and sequential progestogen employ the progestogen for 10–14 days per month (Sturdee *et al.*, 1978). Minimum daily doses of commonly used progestogens are: dydrogesterone 10 mg; levonorgestrel 75 µg; medroxyprogesterone acetate 5 mg; norethisterone 1 mg. In general, doses of progestogen employed have been reduced over the past few years, which has had a beneficial effect on the incidence and severity of symptoms of progestogen intolerance. When such symptoms are troublesome despite low progestogen doses the progestogen course can be cut to only 7 days per month but this does result in a slight increase in cystic hyperplasia.

When hyperplasia does occur in association with HRT many cases can be treated medically. For example, 3 months of treatment with norethisterone 5 mg daily for 3 weeks out of 4 will reverse almost 100% of cases of cystic glandular hyperplasia. Although atypical hyperplasia can, in many cases, be reversed by progestogen, there is a risk that carcinoma may develop despite progestogen treatment. Most clinicians would therefore advise that atypical hyperplasia is an indication for hysterectomy.

Although the addition of cyclical progestogen prevents any excess risk of endometrial carcinoma, unfortunately, it is responsible for the most important clinical complications of HRT, namely the withdrawal bleed and the occurrence of cyclical PMS-like symptoms.

HRT and endometrial cancer

- Do not give oestrogen without accompanying progestogen, to a woman without a uterus
- Ten to fourteen days of progesterone per month protects against endometrial hyperplasia or carcinoma
- Progestogens produce bleeding and PMS-type symptoms

Thrombosis

Recently published data demonstrate that there is a small increase in risk of venous thromboembolism associated with the use of post-menopausal HRT. Three clinical papers were published simultaneously in the *Lancet* in October 1996 (Vandenbroucke, 1996). They used differing methodologies and were related to different populations but all found a slight increase in risk with use of HRT. Their findings have since been confirmed by a large population-based case-control study using the General Practice Research Database in the UK (Guthann *et al.*, 1997).

Overall, the risk of idiopathic venous thromboembolism appears to be doubled by current use of HRT. Importantly, the increased risk appears confined largely to the first year of use. Neither the type, dose nor route of administration appears to influence the risk.

This risk must be put into perspective. The background risk of idiopathic venous thromboembolism among non-users of HRT is about 1.3 per 10 000 women per year. Therefore, use of HRT will result in 1–2 additional cases of venous thromboembolism per 10 000 women per year. This includes both deep vein thrombosis and pulmonary embolism, and fatalities are the exception.

How should these data influence clinical practice? First, women without other risk factors for venous thromboembolism should be advised that the risk is small, and is confined to the first year of use. Secondly, advice should be individualized to put the risk of thromboembolism into the context of a woman's other risk factors for IHD and osteoporosis.

Thirdly, in any woman with a personal history or strong family history of thromboembolism, it would be advisable to obtain the results of a thrombophilia screen prior to initiating HRT. A full screen would include:

- Prothrombin time and activated partial thromboplastin time
- Levels of anti-thrombin 3
- Protein C and protein S
- Activated protein C resistance
- Antiphospholipid antibody and lupus anticoagulant

If any of these tests should prove positive, the advice of a haematologist should be sought as such women may need prophylactic anticoagulation. In women with a relevant history of thromboembolism but a negative thrombophilia screen, it would be prudent to advise a non-oral route of HRT administration (as laboratory data indicate that this may be less thrombogenic than the oral route), and the use of prophylactic low dose aspirin 75 mg daily. The fact that our current tests do not identify an underlying cause does not mean necessarily that there isn't one.

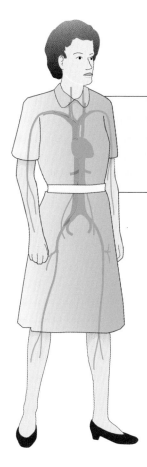

There is a very small increased risk of thromboembolism with the natural oestrogens used in HRT

Breast cancer

The life-time incidence of breast cancer in the developed world is ~10% and any development which may influence this figure warrants careful study. Epidemiological evidence that early menarche, late first pregnancy and late menopause are associated with an increased risk, suggests that post-menopausal oestrogen treatment may similarly increase the risk of breast cancer.

The published data concerning the relationship between HRT and IHD presents a clear message. Unfortunately, interpretation of the research data concerning HRT and breast cancer has not been so clear-cut. A large meta-analysis of 28 studies published in 1991 failed to detect any significant increase in incidence with use of HRT (Dupont and Page, 1991) (Figure 5). Nineteen of the individual studies failed to reach statistical significance, six found an increased incidence and three a reduced incidence. The overall relative risk of breast cancer with oestrogen use was 1.07 but with a non-significant 95% confidence interval of 0.96–1.2. A similar but more selective meta-analysis covering only 16 studies and also published in 1991 did, however, report a significant increase in the incidence of breast cancer with HRT use (Steinberg *et al.*, 1991). The relative risk was 1.3 with a 95% confidence interval of 1.2–1.6.

The most likely reason for this lack of clarity is that breast cancer has a much lower incidence than IHD in post-menopausal women and thus, the majority of studies simply lacked the necessary statistical power to find what they were looking for.

One of the most powerful studies to date that has investigated the effect of HRT on breast cancer risk is the Nurses Health

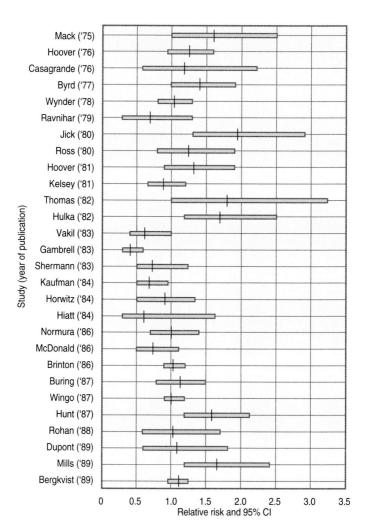

Figure 5
HRT and incidence of breast cancer. CI, confidence interval. [Adapted from
Dupont and Page (1991) with permission.]

Study from the USA. In 1976, 121 700 female registered nurses aged 30–55 were recruited. Baseline information included use of hormones and this information has been updated every 2 years since. The most recent report on breast cancer in this cohort was published in 1995 (Colditz *et al.*, 1995). The results are the most convincing evidence to date of a link between HRT and breast cancer.

Overall, it was found that women currently using oestrogen had a significant increase in the incidence of breast cancer with a relative risk compared to never-users of 1.32 (95% confidence interval, 1.14–1.54). An almost identical increase in incidence was seen in women currently taking oestrogen and progestogen. Thus, the addition of progestogen to oestrogen replacement does not appear to alter the risk of breast cancer.

There was no increase in the incidence of breast cancer in women using HRT who were less than 50 years old. Thus, women who undergo a premature menopause can be reassured that use of HRT until the average age of natural menopause — currently 50 years — carries no increased risk of breast cancer.

The relation between duration of HRT use and breast cancer incidence was interesting. The relative risk increased progressively through 0–2 years and 3–4 years use but did not reach statistical significance until 5 years of use, at which point the relative risk was 1.46 (95% confidence interval, 1.22–1.74). There was no further increase in relative risk with use of HRT extending beyond 10 years.

The age of the woman taking HRT also appeared to have an effect. The incidence of breast cancer increases with advancing age anyway, but older HRT users had a greater risk relative to never-users than younger HRT users.

Any increased risk of breast cancer associated with HRT use disappeared within two years of stopping treatment.

The most recent meta-analysis comes from the Collaborative Group on Hormonal Factors in Breast Cancer (1997). They re-analysed data on 161 316 women from 51 epidemiological studies. Their findings confirm those of the Nurses Health Study that increasing duration of exposure to oestrogen with HRT increases the incidence of breast cancer.

All the above data relates to the incidence of breast cancer. It has previously been thought that the tumours induced by HRT may be of a lower grade with a more benign prognosis than spontaneous breast tumours, leading to the hope that, although the incidence may be increased by HRT, perhaps the mortality would not be. Unfortunately, this appears not to be the case as the Nurses Health Study found that the mortality from breast cancer after 5 or more years of use was significantly raised, to a similar extent as the incidence, with a relative risk of 1.45 (95% confidence interval, 1.01–2.09) (Grodstein *et al.*, 1997). However, all other studies reviewing the mortality have shown a decreased mortality.

HRT and breast cancer risk

- Use of HRT for 5 years or more increases risk of breast cancer
- Mortality may increase similarly
- Risk increases with age and duration of use

In clinical terms a relative risk by itself is of little value. It needs to be applied to the actual risks. The Collaborative Group on Hormonal Factors in Breast Cancer (1997) applied the relative risks derived from their meta-analysis to known age-related incidence rates for breast cancer in the USA and Europe. In women aged between 50 and 70 (compared with never-users of HRT), HRT use for 5 years is associated with a cumulative excess of two breast cancers for every 1000 users. The cumulative excess risk rises to six for every 1000 users with 10 years of HRT use, and to 12 per 1000 users in association with 15 years of HRT use. This must be compared with a cumulative incidence of 45 cases of breast cancer, between ages 50 and 70, per 1000 never-users of HRT. It must be remembered that these predictions of risk relate to women with an average risk of breast cancer. None the less, this method of expressing excess risk is readily understood and may be of use when counselling a woman considering starting HRT.

Genetic predisposition

The issue of genetic predisposition to breast cancer and the relevance of mutations of the BRCA genes is one of the most confusing and rapidly evolving areas of medicine today. Only 1–2% of all breast cancers are thought to be associated with germ-line BRCA mutations. In an individual with one close relative who has had breast cancer diagnosed when more than 50 years old, the chances of her carrying a BRCA1 mutation are only 7%. When more family members have been affected, particularly at an unusually young age, the risks of a mutation increase, perhaps reaching 80% in the case of two close relatives affected when less than 50. However, the place of genetic testing remains highly controversial for a number of reasons. First, there are without doubt predisposing genetic mutations, which have not yet been identified; thus, a negative test may be falsely reassuring. Secondly, there is considerable discrepancy between studies as to the risk of cancer in mutation carriers as the same BRCA1 mutation appears to behave differently in different groups of women. Thirdly, as yet there is no consensus or data on what to do to prevent cancer in an individual identified as at high risk (Healy, 1997).

At the present time, screening for BRCA mutations should not be part of routine clinical practice. Women with one affected family member aged greater than 50 should be reassured that the chance of them carrying an inherited predisposition to breast cancer is small. Most authorities would probably agree that indications for detailed specialist assessment of familial breast cancer risk would include: three or more affected close family members aged greater than 50; two affected relatives aged less than 50; one affected relative aged less than 35 at diagnosis or occurrence of breast cancer in a close male relative.

In practical terms, one cannot counsel a woman regarding the risks and benefits of HRT to her as an individual without taking a full family history enquiring specifically about breast cancer, and then putting the information gathered into the context of our current state of knowledge. Even so, it is not known whether women with a genetic risk or with benign breast disease run any increased risk if given oestrogens.

What of the future? It is hoped that the Selective Estrogen Receptor Modulators (SERMs) such as Raloxifen will offer the benefits of HRT without any increase in risk of breast cancer.

Complications of HRT

The withdrawal bleed

Compliance amongst women taking post-menopausal HRT employing sequentially administered progestogen is poor with only 30% continuing for a year. One of the principal reasons for this is the return of regular withdrawal bleeding. Even if such bleeding is neither heavy, prolonged, painful nor irregular, it is almost invariably a significant nuisance which most post-menopausal women would be happier without. There are several ways in which bleeding can be avoided. Those recommended in current practice are:

Continuous combined HRT

The introduction to general clinical practice of continuous combined regimens of HRT constitutes an important advance. Such regimens combine progestogen with oestrogen continuously and offer the potential to deliver all the benefits of HRT, without periods and without the risk of endometrial carcinoma.

The continuous combination of oestrogen and progestogen results in an atrophic endometrium. Studies of endometrial histology indicate that the endometrium is atrophic in ~90% of women after 3 months of treatment and that this figure rises to nearly 100% after 12 months. The incidence of hyperplasia appears to be low at less than 1%, with very few of these 1% demonstrating atypia. Taking an overview of published data, it appears that 75% of women will be amenorrhoeic after 6 months and that this figure rises to nearer 90% after 12 months (Udoff *et al.*, 1995). The bulk of the remaining women experience only irregular minor spotting. The major drawback is that, in the first 3 months, ~30% of women may experience some heavier and irregular bleeding. Women starting continuous combined HRT should be warned of this possibility and advised if possible to persevere with treatment as in the majority the problem will resolve. When so warned, most women do indeed continue treatment until amenorrhoea is established.

In terms of endometrial safety, the bulk of the data indicates that continuous combined regimens are at least as safe as traditional sequential HRT regimens. However, there have been a handful of reported cases of adenocarcinoma developing. Therefore, it is recommended that resumption of bleeding after established amenorrhoea should always be an indication for endometrial biopsy (Leather *et al.*, 1991). It is concern over endometrial safety that has prompted the recommendation in the data sheets that neither Kliofem nor Premique are to be used within 12 months of the last period.

Perhaps not surprisingly, the absence of uterine bleeding does mean that compliance with continuous combined HRT is much greater than with sequential regimens. A recent study found that after 12 months' treatment with a continuous combined regimen, 97% of women were still on medication, with the figure dropping to 76% at 5 years and 58% at 9 years (Doren and Schneider, 1996). Without any doubt the availability of 'off the shelf' continuous combined preparations (either in tablet form, such as Kliofem and Premique, or as a patch, for example, Evorel Conti) has made continuous combined HRT much easier to prescribe.

Continuous combined HRT

- 75% amenorrhoea at 6 months
- 90% amenorrhoea at 12 months
- 30% irregular bleeding in first 3 months
- 76% remain on treatment at 5 years

Tibolone

The synthetic derivative of norethynodrel which possesses weak oestrogenic, androgenic and progestogenic properties, also offers the prospect of bleeding-free HRT. It has been found to prevent post-menopausal bone loss and to relieve menopausal symptoms. The claim is that it is not uterotrophic, therefore progesterone is unnecessary and there will be no bleeding. Although true for most women, ~15% do experience irregular bleeding. A possible argument against its long-term use is that it may not afford the same protection against IHD as oestrogen because it only possesses weak oestrogenic effects and may reduce HDL cholesterol. Therefore, it is useful for relief of climacteric symptoms where the avoidance of bleeding is of paramount importance because it may result in less breakthrough bleeding than continuous combined oestrogen–progestogen.

Hysterectomy

Hysterectomy should be considered in those women who continue to experience unwanted bleeding despite trying continuous combined HRT. Hysterectomy is the only treatment which guarantees amenorrhoea and it also avoids the need for progestogen therapy of any sort.

Other means of avoiding uterine bleeding are currently available but must be considered inferior to continuous combined HRT, Tibolone or hysterectomy for the following reasons:

Three month cycle sequential HRT

Sequential administration of progestogen once every 3 months has the advantage of only four periods a year. This is still more bleeding than will be experienced with either continuous combined HRT or Tibolone, and there is some data that suggest an increased occurrence of hyperplasia.

Levonorgestrel releasing IUCD

The levonrogestrel releasing IUCD (Mirena) has been used successfully to deliver progestogen to the endometrium in women receiving post-menopausal oestrogen replacement. The incidence of irregular bleeding in the first 3 months of treatment is, however, significantly greater than seen with oral continuous combined HRT, and many women baulk at the idea of a coil in their post-menopausal years.

Unopposed cyclical oestrogens

With the advent of easy to use continuous combined HRT and Tibolone it is very difficult to think of a circumstance in which use of unopposed cyclical oestrogens can be justified.

Endometrial resection

Endometrial ablation either by electroresection or laser cannot currently be recommended. It results in amenorrhoea in only 20% of patients, it does not avoid the need for progestogen and there are no data concerning the long-term effects on bleeding patterns in post-menopausal women using HRT.

Symptoms of progestogen intolerance

The occurrence of unpleasant symptoms during the progestogen course is becoming increasingly recognized as a major problem with sequential oestrogen–progestogen regimes. The range of possible symptoms is wide and resembles very closely those found in pre-menstrual syndrome, the 10 most commonly experienced being: bloating, breast tenderness, mood swings, tiredness, depression, irritability, skin disorders, weight gain, anxiety and generalized aches and pains. Placebo-controlled studies have proven that such symptoms are due to the progestogen content of HRT.

The magnitude of the problem is indicated by one series in which 10% of patients eventually underwent hysterectomy because of progestogenic side effects. The severity of symptoms is related to both the dosage of progestogen and the duration of the cyclical course as well as the type of progestogen used (Smith *et al.*, 1994). In many women, symptoms become particularly severe after the first 7 days of progestogen. Thus, there is a compromise to be reached between avoidance of cystic hyperplasia and minimizing progestogenic symptoms, with 7 days being the shortest permissible progestogen course.

All the currently used progestogens, such as norethisterone, medroxyprogesterone acetate, dydrogesterone and levonorgestrel can cause symptoms, but they may differ in the pattern of symptomatology. Norethisterone appears more likely to give rise to physical symptoms such as headache and tiredness, whereas dydrogesterone has a greater tendency to cause psychological symptoms like depression and irritability. Management of progestogenic symptoms involves reduction in dosage, and shortening of the course together with changing to a different type. Despite these measures many women will choose hysterectomy as a means of continuing to benefit from oestrogen without the problems of cyclical symptoms.

Dependence

In view of the psychoactive properties of oestrogen, in particular the ability to elevate mood, it has been suggested that women receiving HRT may be exhibiting drug dependence, as some women self medicate with greater doses of oral and transdermal oestrogen or request oestradiol implants at decreasing intervals while oestradiol levels are normal or even high. An interesting recent publication found that women on long-term oestrogen implant therapy, who were given placebo implants in a randomized blinded study, experienced more vasomotor symptoms than the women given oestrogen, but did not have any excess of psychological symptoms. There were no signs of a withdrawal syndrome. This evidence is very reassuring that oestrogen treatment is not physically addictive.

The menopause can be considered as a state of hormone deficiency, and HRT is, in effect, merely bringing women back up to the baseline from which they descended as a result. If they are dependent on anything it is the new found good health that HRT brings after years of flushes, sweats, insomnia, fatigue and depression.

Risk/benefit analysis of HRT

At the present time, both the individual woman considering starting HRT, and the physician advising her, are bombarded by the media with a multitude of contradictory messages concerning, on the one hand, the miracle-like benefits of HRT, and on the other, its mortal dangers. It is very important to put these competing risks and benefits into some form of context.

The positive advantages of HRT include: relief of classic menopause symptoms and an increased sense of well-being, which for most women result in improved quality of life, protection from IHD and stroke, prevention of osteoporosis and reduced risk of Alzheimer's disease.

Benefits of HRT

- Relief of menopause symptoms
- Improved quality of life
- 40% reduction in risk of heart disease
- 10% reduction in risk of stroke
- >50% reduction in risk of hip fracture
- Protection from Alzheimer's disease

These benefits of HRT can be difficult to measure. Although none would doubt that oestrogen relieves menopausal vaso-motor symptoms, disease-specific quality of life measures are only now being developed, so any improvement in quality of life is currently difficult to quantify. Similarly, the impact of osteoporosis prevention is difficult to assess. First, mortality from osteoporosis is invariably under-reported in national statistics because many deaths do not immediately follow the fracture and are often attributed to other causes on death certificates. Secondly, osteoporotic spinal disease makes almost no impact on healthcare statistics but is responsible for a vast amount of pain, deformity and disability in older women. Similarly, Alzheimer's disease is rarely mentioned on death certificates, but if the early research suggesting that HRT may offer substantial protection from Alzheimer's is confirmed by others, this will be one of the most attractive benefits of HRT, as it will not only prolong life, but more importantly extend the duration of quality life. This benefit is currently impossible to quantify.

The easiest benefit of HRT to measure is its impact on heart disease. HRT reduces the risk of significant IHD by ~40% and data on heart disease deaths are probably quite accurate. In population terms, IHD is important because it is the leading cause of death amongst women in the post-menopausal years.

The advent of continuous combined HRT and its offer of bleed-free oestrogen replacement means that uterine bleeding

---

Disadvantages of HRT

- Breast cancer risk
- Bleeding
- Progestogen side-effects

---

should no longer be considered a major disadvantage of HRT. This means the only real concern is the risk of breast cancer. On current evidence we must consider that use of HRT may increase the risk of breast cancer, probably by the order of 40% after 10 years of HRT use. This risk is important but must be set against the benefits of HRT. Application of a reduction in death from IHD of 40% and a disputed, slight increase in death from breast cancer to the age-specific mortality rates for these disorders in England and Wales, reveals that the net effect of HRT is a reduced risk of death at all ages (Figure 6). This prediction is borne out by all studies, particularly recently published data from the US Nurses Health Study in which a reduced risk of death was found amongst current HRT users compared with non-users of all ages, and in all previous studies addressing mortality and HRT use. It seems reasonable to conclude that, in strictly numerical terms, a woman is likely to live longer if she uses HRT despite the possible breast cancer risk. If one then considers the impact HRT has on quality of life, the benefits appear even greater.

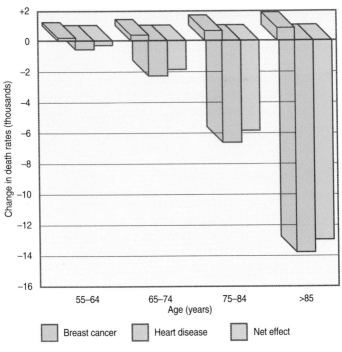

Figure 6
Predicted change in death rates from breast cancer, ischaemic heart disease and the two combined, from use of HRT.

Premature menopause

Menopause occurs prematurely in 1% of women less than 40 years of age. In addition to typical clinical features, the diagnosis must be confirmed by a follicle-stimulating hormone (FSH) >20 IU/l on two or more separate occasions. Ovarian biopsy is never indicated to establish the diagnosis. Resistant ovary syndrome is rare and clinically indistinguishable, but may recover spontaneously with an unexpected return of fertility.

Premature menopause is frequently autoimmune in causation and therefore patients are prone to other autoimmune endocrine disorders.

The tragedy of premature menopause is the unexpected loss of fertility in otherwise healthy young women. This can be treated by assisted conception techniques using donated ova, with excellent results of a 30% pregnancy rate and a 20% live baby rate per cycle.

All the long-term effects of menopause commence at an earlier age and therefore these women are at particular risk of osteoporosis and death from IHD. They are in particular need of HRT, but unfortunately the dose given is usually inadequate to protect the bone and probably equally inadequate for the less easily measured risks of cardiovascular disease. These women need the equivalent of 2 mg of oral 17β-oestradiol daily, a transdermal system delivering 100 μg of oestradiol daily, or replacement with oestrogen implants at 25–50 mg every 6 months depending on the response. Use of HRT in women under the age of 50 does not increase the risk of breast cancer.

Routes of administration of HRT

Three natural oestrogens are commonly used for HRT. 17β-oestradiol is the most commonly used and can be given by mouth, as a percutaneous patch or gel, and as a subcutaneous implant. Conjugated equine oestrogens and oestradiol valerate can only be administered by mouth. Synthetic oestrogens such as mestranol and ethinyloestradiol are not used in HRT and there is no place for the non-steroidal preparation Stilboestrol.

Oral HRT

Oral administration as a tablet has the distinct advantage of being simple and readily acceptable to most women. Furthermore, almost all of the epidemiological data regarding the impact of HRT upon IHD, stroke, thromboembolism and breast cancer has come from the use of oral oestrogen replacement. The oral route does have some disadvantages, however. First, the bulk of any orally ingested oestrogen is converted into oestrone by the gut and liver so that there is a reversal of the normal premenopausal 2:1 ratio of 17β-oestradiol to oestrone. Secondly, oral ingestion produces a first-pass hepatic effect, and thirdly, delivers rapidly a large bolus of oestrogen into the systemic circulation with levels peaking within 4–8 hours and then rapidly declining so that, by 24 hours, levels are little different from baseline. Whether any of these theoretical problems have any clinical significance is unknown.

Non-oral HRT

Non-oral oestrogen delivery, whether by percutaneous patch, gel or subcutaneous implant, avoids many of the theoretical problems of oral therapy mentioned above. Whether avoidance of first-pass hepatic metabolism means that non-oral HRT carries a lower risk of thromboembolism is unproven, but laboratory data suggest that this is likely. Therefore, it seems logical to recommend a non-oral route when giving HRT to an individual at particularly high risk of thrombosis.

The first transdermal oestradiol delivery system, Estraderm TTS, incorporated oestradiol in an alcohol reservoir contained within an adhesive patch. There were problems with skin irritation and poor adhesion. Single membrane patches with the oestrogen contained within the adhesive largely avoid these problems. The first on the market was Evorel, which over the past few years has been joined by several others, including a single membrane version of Estraderm called Estraderm MX. In general, patches need to be changed twice weekly with the exception of FemSeven which lasts 7 days. Adequate replacement usually requires 50–100 µg daily of oestrogen. Skin irritation still occurs but is rarely severe.

Progestogen is also delivered transdermally in Estracombi, but the advantage of this is unclear. The lipid effects of oral progestogen are probably of no clinical significance when given in combination with oestrogen and, because the blood levels of progestogen will need to be the same as obtained with oral progestogen in order to protect the endoemetrium, it seems unlikely that there will be any reduction in adverse progestogenic symptoms.

Oestrogen gels currently available in the UK are Oestrogel and Sandrena. Although some women find it messy, once the gel has been absorbed, which should take no more than 15 minutes, it has all the theoretical advantages of patches without the encumbrance of wearing a patch continuously.

Subcutaneous oestradiol implants offer several advantages over the percutaneous patch. Many women, particularly those who have had a hysterectomy and do not therefore require

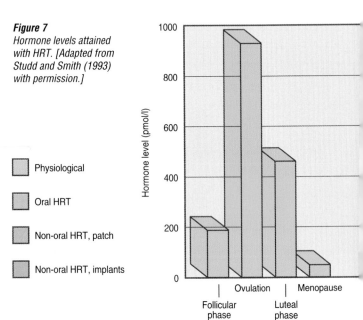

Figure 7
Hormone levels attained with HRT. [Adapted from Studd and Smith (1993) with permission.]

Physiological

Oral HRT

Non-oral HRT, patch

Non-oral HRT, implants

progestogen, find the 6-monthly administration convenient. It is an alternative route of administration for women who experience skin reactions with the patch. Additionally, simultaneous administration of testosterone implants, which are an effective treatment for menopausal primary loss of libido, is easily accomplished. Lastly and most importantly, oestradiol implant therapy is the only route of oestrogen administration which can elevate oestrogen levels back up into the upper premenopausal physiological range. Such levels are important in some women to obtain maximal remedial treatment of osteoporosis and to obtain relief from psychological symptoms.

There are no data to indicate that these higher but still physiological levels are in any way harmful. Long-term implant

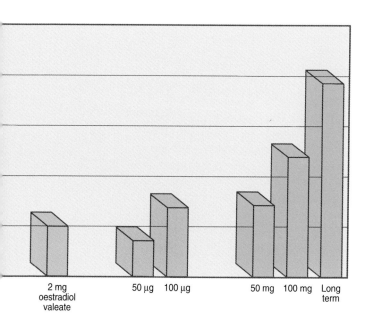

| 2 mg oestradiol valeate | 50 μg | 100 μg | 50 mg | 100 mg | Long term |

therapy achieves average oestradiol levels of 700 pmol/l, roughly intermediate between luteal phase and preovulatory levels. Potential disadvantages of implants are, firstly, that they do have a prolonged duration of action, such that they may still release sufficient oestrogen to produce endometrial stimulation 12–24 months after the last implant. In practice this simply means that when it is desired to discontinue therapy, cyclical progestogen must be continued until it no longer induces a withdrawal bleed.

The other potential problem is that some women may develop supraphysiological oestradiol levels. This so-called tachyphylaxis was only found in 3% of 1388 long-term implant users in one study. Most of these women had been receiving repeat implants at both a higher dose and a shorter interval than recommended, and had a high pre-treatment incidence of psychiatric disorders. It seems that such women with severe PMS or depression require frequent high doses of oestradiol in order to keep symptoms at bay. This may well be a manifestation of a dose–response effect between oestrogen and mood.

In practice, although starting doses may be 50 or 75 mg, eventual maintenance doses should, in general, be 25 or 50 mg every 5–6 months. If used correctly in this manner by a clinician alert to the potential problem, tachyphylaxis should not occur. Where supraphysiological levels already exist, correct management is to continue therapy but at reduced dosage until levels drop back to the physiological range. Complete withdrawal of oestrogen would be both unnecessarily harsh and potentially dangerous.

In addition to treatment of reduced libido, the addition of testosterone implants is highly effective at restoring energy levels and a useful adjunct in the treatment of depression and headaches.

Topical oestrogen

So-called 'local' application of oestrogen to the vagina is used widely. Whilst effective in the relief of vaginal symptoms, there is substantial systemic absorption even when weak oestrogens are administered in low doses, such that endometrial stimulation can occur. Therefore anything but very short-term use must be accompanied by cyclical progestogen.

Practical notes on the prescribing of HRT

Diagnosis of climacteric/menopause

The diagnosis of the menopause is obvious, and identification of the climacteric straightforward, based on a combination of typical symptoms with or without menstrual changes occurring in a woman aged 40–55. Hot flushes, sweats and vaginal dryness are the most reliable symptoms. Increasing frequency or heaviness of periods, or continued menstruation beyond the age of 55 are indications for endometrial biopsy. The diagnosis may be confirmed by an FSH level of >20 IU/l. An FSH of <20 IU/l does not exclude the climacteric, however, as many women experience their most severe symptoms before gonadotrophins are elevated and certainly before their periods stop.

Sometimes increasingly severe PMS symptoms merge with the depression, tiredness and loss of libido of the climacteric. This is often misdiagnosed and badly treated in the premenopausal woman, but usually responds to oestrogen when given in adequate doses.

Investigations

No routine investigations are required before commencing HRT apart from a general examination. A raised FSH may provide confirmatory evidence of the climacteric, and any abnormal bleeding should be investigated. All women should have regular cervical smears, breast examination and mammography, but HRT does not create a need for extra investigations.

Contraindications to HRT

There are very few absolute contraindications to HRT. The orthodox view is that it should not be given to women with recent cancer of the endometrium or breast, although this prohibition may be incorrect. It is said that otosclerosis may deteriorate rapidly during oestrogen therapy but convincing evidence for this view is not available. Most of the contraindications usually listed in data sheets do not apply as they are extrapolations of oral contraceptive data and, while hypertension, hyperlipidaemia and previous coronary thrombosis are contraindications for the oral contraceptive pill, they are indications for HRT.

The presence of IHD or risk factors for IHD should be regarded as positive indications for HRT, because the evidence indicates that HRT reduces substantially the risk of IHD.

A past history of venous thromboembolism should not be regarded as a contraindication to HRT, particularly if the event occurred in association with an obvious precipitant such as pregnancy or post-operatively. In the case of idiopathic or recurrent thrombosis or in the presence of a strong family history a screen for a prothrombotic state should be undertaken. If positive the condition may need treatment in its own right, and the information can be incorporated into the counselling process before commencing treatment.

Progestogens

Women with a uterus must be prescribed progestogen in addition to oestrogen. Ten to fourteen days' progestogen per month is necessary for complete protection of the uterus but women often feel unwell with these tablets with depression, irritability, loss of memory and headaches. Under such circumstances, 7 days may be regarded as a satisfactory compromise in some women. In currently used regimens, progestogens do not appear to alter the cardioprotective effect of oestrogens.

Progestogen is not necessary in women who have had a hysterectomy. It does not protect the breast but often produces cyclical PMS symptoms.

Climacteric women who are still menstruating

It is entirely appropriate to give HRT to symptomatic climacteric women who are still menstruating. It is in the years immediately preceding the cessation of menstruation that symptoms such as depression, irritability and headaches are often most severe. A potential complication is that if the imposed HRT cycle is out of step with the spontaneous ovarian cycle, bleeding problems may ensue with the woman having two periods each month. In women with a 28-day cycle, this is avoided easily by always commencing combined preparations on the first day of a period, or when prescribing separately, by ensuring that progestogen is given always in what would be the luteal phase of the spontaneous cycle. Alternatively, the dose of percutaneous oestrogen can be increased until spontaneous ovarian function is suppressed. This is not so easy to achieve with oral oestrogen. If cycle control is not rapidly obtained, even in a woman who had a previously normal bleeding pattern, the endometrium should be biopsied. A good 'off the shelf' preparation is Femoston 2/10.

The management of bleeding problems on HRT

The majority of women receiving continuous oestrogen and cyclical progestogen will have regular withdrawal bleeds. Up to 5%, however, will be amenorrhoeic particularly when the dose of oestrogen is low and that of progestogen relatively high. Such amenorrhoea is not an indication for endometrial biopsy. It occurs because the proliferative action of oestrogen is being inhibited completely by the progestogen.

The withdrawal bleed should start 1–5 days after the end of the progestogen course. The premature onset of bleeding whilst still taking progestogen suggests that full secretory transformation of the endometrium is not occurring and indicates the need for more progestogen. The first step is to increase the duration of the progestogen course to a maximum of 14 days. If the problem is not corrected then the dose should be increased. If the problem persists despite these measures the endometrium should be biopsied.

Any other pattern of abnormal bleeding also requires biopsy. This includes any persistent increase in menstrual flow, and any irregular bleeding. The majority of endometrial biopsies can be performed as an outpatient procedure using either a Pipelle or Vabra aspiration. In most cases, cystic glandular hyperplasia can be reversed with a 3-month course of norethisterone 5 mg, three times a day, for 3 out of every 4 weeks. If the subsequent biopsy is then normal the patient must be maintained on a full 14 day per month cyclical regime preferably with norethisterone 5 mg daily. In the presence of atypical hyperplasia, hysterectomy is the best course of action.

In the presence of normal endometrial histology, continuous combined HRT may be a means of controlling bleeding in some cases.

Despite manipulating progestogen there will be a significant number of women who have persistent troublesome bleeding with normal endometrial histology. There is a much greater place for hysterectomy in such women than is currently realised. In experienced hands the procedure is safe; it guarantees amenorrhoea and completely avoids the need for progestogen. In women with severe bleeding problems, it should be considered by the physician and offered sooner rather than later in order to avoid years of unnecessary menstrual misery. With modern surgical techniques, the uterus can be removed vaginally without the need for potentially dangerous and scarring laparoscopic assistance, and with the ability to offer the individual woman the choice as to whether she keeps her ovaries and/or cervix.

Hysterectomy
• Amenorrhoea guaranteed
• Avoids need for progestogen
• Vaginal route has low morbidity, rapid recovery and no scarring
• Can retain or remove ovaries and/or cervix
• Vaginal surgery is a minimal access procedure

The use of endometrial ablative techniques cannot be recommended. Their use results in a high incidence of post-operative dysmenorrhoea and the operation does not obviate the need for continuing use of cyclical progestogen. Even if amenorrhoea results there are still islands of hormone-responsive endometrium remaining in the uterus which could theoretically undergo malignant change if unopposed oestrogens were used.

HRT in women with a past history of breast or endometrial cancer

This is a complex and emotive issue. Many clinicians instinctively take the view that, once breast cancer is diagnosed, HRT should be stopped and not used again in that individual under any circumstances, for fear that its use will increase dramatically the risk and rate of progress of recurrent cancer. Whilst this view is entirely understandable it is not supported by what scant data there is. There is now a handful of published series of women who have used HRT after a diagnosis of breast cancer. In all these series, the numbers are small and the women were not randomized; they suggest that recurrence is not increased after HRT use. One US series followed 77 women who used HRT after treatment for breast cancer. After a median follow up of 5 years (range, 10 months to 35 years), seven women had developed recurrent cancer, whilst 70 were disease free (DiSaia et al., 1993). No one would interpret these data as indicating that HRT carries no risk in breast cancer survivors. It seems reasonable that if a strong indication for HRT exists, an individual woman should be given the choice to take oestrogen. This comes down to a quality of life issue. Some women will consider an unquantifiable increase in the risk of recurrent breast cancer is justified by the improved sense of well-being and quality of life that is brought by HRT.

It would be reasonable to consider use of HRT under the following circumstances:

> (i) When there is a high chance that initial treatment has been curative (small tumour, nodes free, histologically non-aggressive).
>
> (ii) When a disease-free survival over several years indicates only a small risk of secondary disease.
>
> (iii) When menopausal symptoms are so bad as to severely reduce the quality of life.
>
> (iv) When the bone density is dangerously low.

Each case must be considered individually on its merits and the potential risks and benefits discussed fully with the patient.

Endometrial cancer which is considered to be cured, by virtue of being an early stage, well differentiated and node-negative, need not be considered a contraindication to HRT.

HRT in the over 60s

The indications for HRT are, if anything, even stronger in the older woman in whom the risks of heart disease and stroke are greater. HRT in these patients results in the same improvements in bone density, energy and well-being as are seen in younger women. Age must not be a barrier to HRT.

Contraception

The BNF currently warns that a woman should be considered potentially fertile for 2 years after her last period if aged under

50 and for 1 year after her last period if over 50. In practical terms, a woman with menopausal symptoms and an FSH greater than 40 IU/l is extremely unlikely to conceive.

When the FSH is between 15 and 40 IU/l some primordial follicles may persist so that further episodes of spontaneous ovarian activity may occur. The dose of oestrogen in most HRT preparations will not be sufficient to suppress ovarian activity. Therefore, if conception is not desired, some form of contraception should be advised.

Women with apparent premature menopause must be warned that occasionally ovarian function can return and ovulation occur. Although this is very unlikely, the possibility must be borne in mind and women counselled accordingly.

Choice of preparation

For most women, the initial choice will be between oral therapy and patch therapy. The convenience of the 'off the shelf' preparations combining oestrogen and progestogen in the same pack means that one of these should be tried initially. There is an almost bewildering variety of preparations currently available. In general terms, a preparation containing a higher dose of oestrogen, such as 2 mg daily orally, or a patch delivering 50–100 ug daily, should be chosen. Certainly higher oestrogen doses will have a greater beneficial impact on bone density and protection from osteoporosis. Higher oestrogen levels also appear more effective in relieving psychological symptoms.

Whether transdermal or oral HRT is better is unknown. It is fair to say that the bulk of the data on which our knowledge of HRT is derived from use of oral HRT. Therefore, perhaps oral HRT should be the first choice. In perimenopausal women, progestogen should be added sequentially. In post-menopausal women, we should probably now recommend continuous combined therapy given the far better compliance achieved when there is no uterine bleeding.

Subcutaneous implants of oestrogen should be considered in women known to have particularly poor bone density, and in women whose symptoms fail to respond to oral or patch therapy. In both these circumstances, the advantage of implants is the higher level of oestradiol achieved.

Relative potency of oestrogens

Low	Medium	High	Very High
Conjugated oestrogens 0.625 µg	Conjugated oestrogens 1.25 µg	Patch 100 µg oestradiol daily	Oestradiol implant 100 mg decreases to 50 mg long term
Oestradiol 1 mg	Oestradiol 2 µg	Oestradiol implant 50 mg decreasing to 25 mg long term	
Patch delivery 25 µg oestradiol daily	Patch delivery 50 µg oestradiol daily		

Table 1

Progestogen should always be prescribed together with oestrogen in a woman with a uterus.

Progestogen is not necessary in a woman who has had a hysterectomy and oestrogen replacement can be given alone.

Duration of HRT

HRT should be continued for at least 5 years beyond the average age of menopause if it is to confer appreciable protection against osteoporosis. In practice this means at least until 55 years of age. The degree of protection will be even greater the longer HRT is continued beyond this age. The same applies to protection from heart disease. It is only current HRT use which confers protection, and the incidence of cardiovascular disease increases exponentially with age. Adding to this the probability that HRT protects from Alzheimer's disease, then one has powerful evidence to advise women to continue HRT use into old age in order to gain maximum benefit. The only down side is the fear of breast cancer, but the overall risk–benefit analysis means that the above benefits outweigh the possible breast cancer risks.

Counselling

In an ideal world, all women should be seen by an interested informed physician as they enter the menopausal transition. They should be given information, and advice should be tailored to the unique circumstances of the individual. The most appropriate person to fulfil this role is the family doctor, but with the support of an expert when necessary. This is a confusing field. The physician's task is to ensure as far as possible that women are empowered to make truly informed choices about HRT, and not be frightened or lured into an inappropriate decision by media sensationalism.

References

Brincat M, Moniz CF, Studd JWW, Darby A, Magos A, Emburey G and Versi E (1985) Long-term effect of the menopause and sex hormones on skin thickness. *Br J Obstet Gynaecol*, **92**: 256–259.

Bungay GT, Vessey MP and McPherson CK (1980) Study of symptoms in middle life with special reference to menopause. *Br Med J*, **ii**: 181–183.

Bush TL, Barrett-Cvonnor E and Cowan LD (1987) Cardiovascular mortality and non-contraceptive use of estrogen in women: results from the lipid research clinics program follow-up study. *Circulation*, **75**: 1102–1109.

Cardozo LD and Kelleher C (1997) Lower urinary tract dysfunction and the menopause. In *Urogynaecology*. L Cardozo (ed), Churchill Livingstone, London, pp. 443–460.

Christiansen C and Christiansen MS (1981) Bone mass in postmenopausal women after withdrawal of oestrogen/gestagen therapy. *Lancet*, **i**: 459–461.

Colditz GA, Hankinson SE, Hunter DJ, Willett WC, Manson JE, Stampfer MJ, Hennekens C, Rosner B and Speizer FE (1995) The use of estrogens and progestins and the risk of breast cancer in postmenopausal women. *N Engl J Med*, **332**: 1589–1593.

Collaborative Group on Hormonal Factors in Breast Cancer (1997) Breast cancer and hormone replacement therapy: collaborative reanalysis of data from 51 epidemiological studies of 52 705 women with breast cancer and 108 411 women without breast cancer. *Lancet*, **350**: 1047–1059.

Darling GM, Johns JA, McCloud PI and Davis SR (1997) Estrogen and progestin compared with simvastatin for hypercholesterolaemia in postmenopausal women. *N Engl J Med*, **337**: 595–601.

Ditkoff EC, Crary WG, Cristo M and Lobo RA (1991) Estrogen improves psychological function in asymptomatic postmenopausal women. *Obstet Gynecol*, **78**: 991–995.

DiSaia PJ, Odicono F, Grosen EA, Cowan B, Pecorelli S and Wile AG (1993) Hormone replacement therapy in breast cancer. *Lancet*, **342**: 1232.

Doren M and Schneider HP (1996) Long-term compliance of continuous combined estrogen and progestogen replacement in postmenopausal women. *Maturitas*, **25**: 99–105.

Dupont WD and Page DL (1991) Menopausal estrogen replacement therapy and breast cancer. *Arch Int Med*, **151**: 67–72.

Gregoire AJP, Kumar R, Everitt B, Henderson AF and Studd JWW (1996) Transdermal oestrogen for the treatment of severe postnatal depression. *Lancet*, **347**: 930–933.

Grodstein F, Stampfer MJ, Colditz GA, Willett WC, Manson JE, Joffe M, Rosner B, Fuchs C, Hankinson SE, Hunter DJ, Hennekens CH and Speizer FE (1997) Postmenopausal hormone therapy and mortality. *N Engl J Med*, **336**: 1769–1775.

Gutthann SP, Rodriguez LAG, Castellsague J and Oliart AD (1997) Hormone replacement therapy and risk of venous thromboembolism: population based case-control study. *Br Med J*, **314**: 796–800.

Healy B (1997) BRCA genes — bookmaking, fortunetelling, and medical care. *N Engl J Med*, **336**: 1448–1449.

Hunt K, Vessey M and McPherson K (1990) Mortality in a cohort of long-term users of hormone replacement therapy: an updated analysis. *Br J Obstet Gynaecol*, **97**: 1080–1086.

Kannus P, Parkkari J and Niemi S (1995) Age-adjusted incidence of hip fractures. *Lancet*, **346**, 50–51.

Karpf DB, Shapiro DR, Seeman E, Ensrud KE, Johnston CC, Jr, Adami S, Harris ST, Santora AC, II, Hirsch LJ, Oppenheimer L and Thompson D (1997) Prevention of nonvertebral fractures by Alendronate. *JAMA*, **277(14)**: 1159–1164.

Keil DP, Felson DT, Anderson JJ, Wilson DWF and Moskowitz MA (1987) Hip fractures and use of oestrogens in postmenopausal women. *N Engl J Med*, **317**: 1169–1174.

Klaiber EL, Broverman DM, Vogel W and Kobayashi Y (1979) Estrogen replacement therapy for severe persistent depression in women. *Arch Gen Psych*, **36**: 550–554.

Leather AT, Sarras M and Studd JW (1991) Endometrial histology and bleeding patterns after eight years of continuous combined oestrogen and progestogen therapy in post-menopausal women. *Obstet Gynaecol*, **78(6)**: 1008–1010.

Lindsay R, Hart DM, Aitken JM, McDonald EB, Andersen JB and Clare AC (1976) Long-term prevention of postmenopausal osteoporosis by oestrogen. *Lancet*, **i**: 1038–1040.

McKinley SM and Jefferys M (1974) The menopausal syndrome. *Br J Prev Soc Med*, **28**: 108–115.

Montgomery JC, Appleby L, Brincat M, Versi E, Tapp A, Fenwick PBC and Studd JWW (1987) Effect of oestrogen and testosterone implants on psychological disorders in the climacteric. *Lancet*, **i**: 297–299.

Office of Population Censuses and Statistics Cause (1993) Series DH2, No.20. London: HMSO, 1994.

Paganini-Hill A, Ross RK and Henderson BE (1988) Postmenopausal oestrogen treatment and stroke: a prospective study. *Br Med J*, **297**: 519–522.

Porter M, Penney GC, Russell D, Russell E and Templeton A (1996) A population based survey of women's experience of menopause. *Br J Obstet Gynaecol*, **103**: 1025–1028.

Smith RNJ, Holland EFN and Studd JWW (1994) The symptom-atology of progestogen intolerance. *Maturitas*, **18**: 87–91.

Smith RNJ and Studd JWW (1994) Estrogens and depression in women. In *Treatment of the postmenopausal woman*. RA Lobo (ed), Raven Press, New York, pp. 129–136.

Smith RNJ, Studd JWW, Zamblera D and Holland EFN (1995) A randomised comparison over 8 months of 100 µg and 200 µg twice weekly doses of transdermal oestradiol in the treatment of severe premenstrual syndrome. *Br J Obstet Gynaecol*, **102**: 475–484.

Stampfer MJ and Colditz GA (1991) Estrogen replacement therapy and coronary heart disease: a quantitative assessment of the available evidence. *Prev Med*, **20**: 47–63.

Steinberg KK, Thacker SB and Smith SJ (1991) A meta-analysis of the effect of estrogen therapy on breast cancer. *JAMA*, **265**: 1985–1990.

Stevenson JC and Whitehead M (1982) Postmenopausal osteoporosis. *Br Med J*, **285**: 585–588.

Stevenson JC, Cust MP, Gangar KF, Hillard TC, Lees B and Whitehead MI (1990) Effects of transdermal versus oral hormone replacement therapy on bone density in spine and proximal femur in postmenopausal women. *Lancet*, **336**: 265–269.

Studd JWW and Smith RNJ (1993) Oestradiol and testosterone implants in menopause management. *Bailliere's Clin Endocrinol Metab*, **7**: 203–224.

Studd JWW and Smith RNJ (1994) Oestrogens and depression. *Menopause*, **1**: 33–37.

Studd JWW, Savvas M, Watson N, Garnett T, Fogelman I and Cooper D (1990) The relationship between plasma estradiol and the increase in bone density in postmenopausal women after treatment with subcutaneous hormone implants. *Am J Obstet Gynecol*, **163**: 1474–1479.

Sturdee DW, Wade-Evans T, Paterson MEL, Thom M and Studd JWW (1978) Relations between bleeding pattern, endometrial histology and oestrogen treatment in menopausal women. *Br Med J*, **i**: 1575.

Tang M-X, Jacobs D, Stern Y, Marder K, Schofield P, Gurland B and Andrews H (1996) Effect of oestrogen during menopause on risk and age at onset of Alzheimer's disease. *Lancet*, **348**: 429–432.

Udoff L, Langenberg P and Adashi EY (1995) Combined continuous hormone replacement therapy: a critical review. *Obstet Gynecol*, **86**: 306–316.

Vandenbroucke JP and Helmerhorst FM (1996) Risk of venous thromboembolism with hormone replacement therapy. *Lancet*, **348**: 972.

Index

Aches and pains, 9
Adenocarcinoma, 33
Age, and HRT, 54
Alcohol, skin patches, 43
Alendronate, 14
Alzheimer's disease,
    20–1, 38, 57
Amenorrhoea, 33, 34,
    35, 51, 52, 53
Androgen deficiency,
    and loss of libido,
    8–9
Andropatch, 9
Angina, 19–20
Arteries, 18
Aspirin, 25
Atherosclerosis, 18
Atrophy:
    generalized, 9
    urogenital, 5
Autoimmune disorders,
    40

Biopsy, endometrial, 22,
    48, 50, 51
Bisphosphates, 14
Bleeding:
    abnormal, 48, 49, 51
    management of
        bleeding problems,
        51–3
    menstruation, 48, 50
    withdrawal bleed, 23,
        32–4, 51
Bone:
    density scans, 13
    see also Osteoporosis

Breasts:
    cancer, 26–31, 39, 41,
        49, 53–4, 57
    examinations, 49
    mammography, 49

Calcitonin, 13
Calcium, 13
Cancer:
    adenocarcinoma, 33
    breast, 26–31, 39, 41,
        49, 53–4, 57
    endometrial, 21–2, 49,
        53, 54
Candidiasis, 5
Cervical smears, 49
Cholesterol, 18
Climacteric:
    definition, 1
    diagnosis, 48
    HRT during, 50–1
Clonidine, 4
Collagen, 9
Complications of HRT,
    32–41
Concentration problems,
    6
Confidence, loss of, 5–6
Connective tissue,
    atrophy, 9
Continuous combined
    HRT, 56
    and heart disease, 19
    and withdrawal
        bleeding, 32–4, 52
Contraception, 54–5
Contraceptive pill, 49

Contraindications, 49–50
Coronary heart disease
    see Ischaemic
    heart disease
Counselling, 57
Crush fractures, 10
Cystitis, 5

Death rates:
    breast cancer, 29, 39,
        40
    heart disease, 14–15,
        40
    risk/benefit analysis,
        38–40
Deep vein thrombosis, 24
Depression, 1, 5–8, 37
    in climacteric, 50
    dydrogesterone and, 36
    oestradiol and, 46
    progestogen and, 50
    testosterone and, 47
Dydrogesterone, 22, 36
Dysmenorrhoea, 53
Dyspareunia, 5

Endometrium:
    ablation, 35, 53
    biopsy, 22, 48, 50, 51
    cancer, 21–2, 23, 49,
        53, 54
    continuous combined
        HRT, 32–3
    hyperplasia, 22, 32–3,
        51
    oestrogen implants and,
        46

Estracombi, 43
Estraderm, 43
Ethinyloestradiol, 42
Etidronate, 14
Evorel, 43

Fainting, 4
Femoral neck fractures,
    10–11, 13
Femoston 2/10, 51
FemSeven, 43
Fluoride, 13
Follicle-stimulating
    hormone (FSH),
    49, 55
Fractures, 10, 11, 13, 14,
    38

Gels, 43, 44
Genetics, and breast
    cancer, 30–1
Genital atrophy, 5
Giddiness, 4
Gonadotrophins, 1, 3, 4,
    48

Headaches, 4, 8
    in climacteric, 50
    norethisterone and, 36
    progestogen and, 50
    testosterone and, 47
Heart disease see
    Ischaemic heart
    disease
High-density lipoprotein
    (HDL), 18, 19
Hip fractures, 10–11, 13
Hormone replacement
    therapy (HRT):
    complications, 32–41
    contraindications, 49
    dosages, 4
    duration, 57
    numbers using, 2
    in the over 60s, 54
    risk/benefit analysis,
        37–9
    see also Oestrogen;
        Progestogen
Hot flushes, 1, 3, 4, 37,
    48
Hypercholesterolaemia,
    19
Hyperlipidaemia, 17,
    19–20, 49

Hypertension, 19–20, 49
Hysterectomy, 22, 34,
    36, 45, 50, 52

Implants, 37, 41, 43,
    45–6, 56
Insomnia, 3, 4, 6, 37
Investigations, 49
Irritability, 5–6, 36, 50
Ischaemic heart disease
    (IHD), 14–19
    duration of HRT, 57
    as indication for HRT,
        49
    oestrogen and, 39
    in the over 60s, 54
    premature menopause,
        41
    incidence with HRT,
        15–16
    mortality rates, 14–15
    oestrogen and, 15–18,
        19
    progestogen and,
        18–19
IUCDs, levonorgestrel-
    releasing, 35

Kliofem, 33

Levonorgestrel, 22, 36
Levonorgestrel releasing
    IUCDs, 35
Libido, loss of, 5, 6, 8–9,
    45
Lipids, 18–19
Low-density lipoprotein
    (LDL), 18, 19

Mammography, 49
Medroxyprogesterone
    acetate, 22, 36
Memory loss, 6, 20, 50
Menopause:
    definition, 1
    diagnosis, 48
    premature, 40–1
    symptoms, 3–9
Menstruation, 48, 50
Mestranol, 42
Mirena, 35
Muscles, aches and
    pains, 9
Myocardial infarction,
    19–20

Neurotransmitters, 20
Night sweats, 1, 3, 4, 6,
    37, 48
Non-oral HRT, 43–7
Norethisterone, 22, 36,
    51
Norethynodrel, 34

Oestradiol, 42
    implants, 37, 45–6, 56
    and osteoporosis, 13
    for premature
        menopause, 41
    and psychological
        symptoms, 7
Oestro-gel, 44
Oestrogen:
    and Alzheimer's
        disease, 20–1
    and breast cancer,
        26–31, 53–4
    choice of preparation,
        55–6
    continuous combined
        HRT, 32–4
    contraindications, 49
    dependence on, 36–7
    effects on skin, 9
    endometrial hyperplasia
        and carcinoma,
        21–2
    falling levels, 1
    and ischaemic heart
        disease, 15–18, 19,
        39
    non-oral administration,
        43–7
    oral administration,
        42–3
    and osteoporosis,
        11–13
    for premature
        menopause, 41
    and psychological
        symptoms, 7–8
    relative potency, 56
    risk/benefit analysis,
        37–9
    and stroke risk, 17
    topical oestrogen, 47
    unopposed cyclical
        oestrogens, 35
    and vasomotor
        symptoms, 4
    withdrawal bleeding, 51

Oestrone, 42
Oral HRT, 42–3, 55–6
Osteoporosis, 10–14, 38, 55
  bone loss, 1
  duration of HRT, 57
  fluoride and, 13
  oestradiol implants, 45
  premature menopause, 41
Otosclerosis, 49
Ovaries, 55
  failure of, 1, 3
  hysterectomy, 52
  premature menopause, 40

Patches, 43–4, 55
Percutaneous patches, 43–4
Polycystic ovary syndrome, 11
Post-natal depression, 6
Pre-menstrual syndrome (PMS), 6, 23, 46, 48, 50
Premarin, 18, 19
Premature menopause, 11, 40–1, 55
Premique, 33
Progestogen:
  and breast cancer, 28
  choice of preparation, 55–6
  continuous combined HRT, 32–4
  dosage, 50
  and endometrial carcinoma, 23
  and endometrial hyperplasia, 22

and ischaemic heart disease, 18–19
and oestradiol implants, 46
side-effects, 35–6
three month cycle sequential HRT, 35
transdermal patches, 44
and vaginal oestrogens, 47
and vasomotor systems, 4
withdrawal bleeding, 51
Provera, 19
Psychological symptoms, 5–8, 45, 55
Pulmonary embolism, 24

Raloxifen, 31
Resistant ovary syndrome, 40
Risk/benefit analysis, 37–9

Salpingo-oopherectomy, 36
Selective Estrogen Receptor Modulators (SERMs), 31
Simvastin, 19
Skin, thinning, 1, 9
Skin patches, 43–4, 55
Sleep disturbances, 3, 4, 6, 37
Stilboestrol, 42
Stroke, 17, 54
Sweats, 1, 3, 4, 6, 37, 48

Tachyphylaxis, 46

Testosterone, 8–9, 45, 47
Thombosis, 49
Three month cycle sequential HRT, 35
Thrombosis, 23–5, 43
Tibolone, 34
Tiredness, 36, 37
Transdermal patches, 44

Urinary symptoms, 5
Uterus:
  endometrial carcinoma, 21–2, 23
  endometrial hyperplasia, 22, 32–3
  hysterectomy, 22, 34, 36, 45, 50, 51, 52
  levonorgestrel releasing IUCDs, 35
  progestogen therapy, 49–50
  withdrawal bleeding, 32–4

Vagina:
  dryness, 1, 3, 4, 5, 48
  `local' application of oestrogen, 43
Vasomotor symptoms, 4, 37
Vertebral crush fractures, 10

Withdrawal bleeding, 23, 32–4, 51